Summary

Of

The Real Anthony Fauci:

Bill Gates, Big Pharma, and the Global War on
Democracy and Public Health

(Children's Health Defense)

By

Robert F. Kennedy Jr.

Jesse Labon

TABLE OF CONTENTS

4

INTRODUCTION

Robert F. Kennedy Jr.'s book The Real Anthony Fauci uncovers how "America's Doctor" got his start in the early days of the AIDS crisis by working with pharmaceutical companies to destroy safe and effective off-patent AIDS therapies.

The book was written to raise awareness about Anthony Fauci's role in allowing pharmaceutical companies to have control over our government.

It explains how Fauci, Gates, and others wield control over the media, scientific journals, key government and quasi-governmental agencies, global intelligence agencies, and influential scientists and physicians to inundate the public with fearful propaganda about COVID-19 virulence and pathogenesis, as well as silence debate and censor dissent.

The corporate media, which is funded by the pharmaceutical industry, has persuaded millions of Americans that Dr. Anthony Fauci is a hero.

Dr. Anthony Fauci, the director of the National Institute of Allergy and Infectious Diseases (NIAID), is in charge of disbursing $6.1 billion in taxpayer-funded scientific research each year, giving him complete control over the subject, content, and outcome of scientific health research all over the world.

Dr. Anthony Fauci, as you may know, was the most powerful and long-serving public health officer in the United States. He was involved in the planning and execution of the historic coup against Western democracy. His narrative has never been shared, and those in power have fought tooth and nail to keep it hidden. In 16 comparable countries, the average decline in life expectancy was 1.9 years in the United States. Each month, 10,000 children die as a result of global lockdowns caused by virus-related starvation.

Over the next 15 years, unemployment shock is anticipated to result in an extra 890,000 fatalities. Dr. Anthony Fauci is the world's most powerful and tyrannical doctor. He put pharmaceutical profits and personal benefit ahead of public health and safety. A recent book, Dr. Phauci's Pharmanation, details his abuse of hundreds of Black and Hispanic orphans and foster children.

As the trusted public face of the US government's reaction to COVID, Dr. Anthony Fauci sold the American public on a new destiny. The author's family has had a strong association with America's public health bureaucracy for the past 80 years. He stood by and watched as industry used indentured slaves on Capitol Hill to empty out agencies that were supposed to be under control. As a result, Congress established sock puppets to govern the very business it was supposed to regulate.

Bob Greene has fought the US Environmental Protection Agency (EPA) and other environmental agencies for four decades in an attempt to expose and remedy the corrupt sweetheart deals that put regulators in bed with the polluting corporations they were supposed to regulate. Greene: The web of entanglements between pharmaceutical firms and government-run health agencies had pushed regulatory capture to unprecedented heights.

During the 2020 COVID-19 pandemic, Dr. Anthony Fauci was at the center of a global drama unlike any other in human history. The horrifying story that unfolds here has never been told before, and many people in positions of power have tried tirelessly to keep the public in the dark.

Dr. Anthony Fauci's calm, authoritative, and amiable manner was Prozac for Americans terrified by two existential crises, the Trump presidency and COVID-19. On the White House stage, his calm, steady presence gave Democrats and idealistic liberals hope.

Dr. Tony Fauci's charisma and commanding voice won him widespread, if not universal, appreciation. Frida Ghitis believes he campaigned for both his own canonization and an unnerving inquisition against dissenters. Science, she maintains, thrives on skepticism of official orthodoxies.

Dr. Anthony Fauci enjoys this degree of admiration from the world's finest doctors due to his direct and indirect control over 57 percent of global biomedical research funding. He has the power to shape and sustain the prevailing global medical narratives, as well as to reinforce the assumption that he is the embodiment of science. Surgeon General Tony Fauci's 50-year tenure has proven terrible for both public health and democracy. His botched management of the COVID outbreak was also a disaster. The United States accounted for 14.5 percent of all COVID deaths, while having only 4% of the world's population.

Dr. Anthony Fauci's prescriptions are frequently more lethal than the ailments they are designed to treat. His COVID medicines were also ineffective. According to the findings, during the quarantine, life expectancy dropped by 1.9 years. Millions of people have died as a result of unemployment, delayed medical care, despair, obesity, stress, overdoses, suicide, addiction, alcoholism, and accidents. Between 2018 and 2020, the average life expectancy at birth in the United States decreased by 1.9 years.

Some of the things you'll learn from this book include:

Quarantine Caused Deaths

There was an 8.5-fold increase over the average drops in 16 comparable countries. We haven't seen something like this since World War II.

300 million people become destitute, food insecure, and hungry. By 2020, disruptions in health and nutrition services will have killed 228,000 children in South Asia. Unemployment shock is expected to result in an additional 890,000 deaths over the next 15 years. One-third of teens and young adults stated their mental health had deteriorated throughout the pandemic. Overdose deaths in the United States increased by 30% in 2020, to 93,000.

Overdoses from synthetic opioids increased by 38.4%. In June 2020, 11% of adults in the United States were contemplating suicide.

Economic Destruction and Wealth Redistribution

During the COVID pandemic, Dr. Anthony Fauci was the ringmaster in the premeditated destruction of America's economy. His lockdown wreaked havoc on the country's once-thriving economic engine. Government officials have already begun liquidating the New Deal's legacies.

Increasing the Wealth of the Wealthy

Dr. Anthony Fauci's business closures destroyed America's middle class, resulting in the largest upward transfer of wealth in human history. The biggest winners were the behemoths of Big Technology, Big Data, Big Telecom, Big Finance, and Big Media.

Robber barons quickly transformed America's democracy into a surveillance police state using technology, data, and telecommunications. These corporations backed up all official declarations, while stifling any opposition. Mark Zuckerberg, Sergey Brin, and Jeff Bezos all saw their fortunes increase by $35 billion, $41 billion, and $86 billion, respectively.

Ellison, Gates, and others took advantage of the shutdown to hasten the creation of their 5G network of satellites, antennae, biometric facial recognition, and track-and-trace equipment, which they and their government and spy agency partners may use to collect and monetize our data.

While the outlaw gang destroyed our democracy, civil rights, country, and way of life, we huddled in organized panic from a flu-like sickness. And we were informed that it would just be for 15 days, or possibly 15 months, or however long Dr. Fauci decides to evaluate the data.

Upward Failing

The public's health has worsened substantially under Dr. Anthony Fauci's half-century as director of the National Institute of Allergy and Infectious Diseases. The generation born after his accession is the sickest in the history of the United States. The United States has the poorest health-care system among industrialized nations, with the highest infant mortality and life expectancy.

When Dr. Tony Fauci took head the National Institute of Allergy and Infectious Diseases in 1984, 12.8 percent of children had allergic, autoimmune, or chronic illnesses. 80 autoimmune diseases, including juvenile diabetes and rheumatoid arthritis, were almost unknown until 1984.

170 illnesses became widespread in the late 1980s, after vaccine manufacturers were granted government immunity against lawsuits. Processed foods, corn syrup, and PFOA flame retardants could all play a role. Tony Fauci has shown little interest in funding basic research to address these problems.

Pharmacology of Dr. Phauci

Dr. Anthony Fauci's failure to accomplish public health goals during the COVID outbreak is not a single episode, but rather part of a trend of prioritizing pharmaceutical profits and self-interest before public health and safety. Anthony Fauci's two-decade drive to promote bogus pandemics as a vehicle to market new vaccinations, drugs, and pharmaceutical businesses, his atrocities against hundreds of Black and Hispanic orphans and foster children, whom he subjected to severe and death medical testing.

As I previously indicated, Robert F. Kennedy's book, The Real Anthony Fauci, was written in order to inform Americans about Anthony Fauci's sinister role in helping pharmaceutical companies to exert control over our government. That is also the purpose of this summary.

Happy reading!

CHAPTER ONE

Mismanaging A Pandemic

Arbitrary Decrees: Science-Free Medicine

Dr. Anthony Fauci's technique of mandatory masking, social separation, and quarantining the healthy (also known as lockdowns) was used to handle the COVID-19 pandemic. This strategy of containing an infectious disease outbreak has never been used in public health before, and it was based on shaky scientific basis. "There is absolutely no reason to wear a mask," Dr. Anthony Fauci said in January. Regular masking (wearing less than a N95 respirator) has little influence on viral infection rates in hospitals and operating rooms, according to peer-reviewed research. Dr. Anthony Fauci's decision to support masks after earlier rejecting them came at a time when political division was at an all-time high, and masks quickly became important tribal symbols.

The psychological effects of disguise reminded me of my "duck and cover" training as a kid. Dr. Anthony Fauci and other officials did not do any research or make any statements regarding whether lockdowns would cause more injury or death than they prevented. COVID infections and mortality do not differ much between counties that require severe lockdowns and masks and those that do not.

Noble Lies and Bad Data

According to the New York Times, Dr. Anthony Fauci's estimate of vaccine coverage needed to establish "herd immunity" has risen from 70% in March to 80–90% in September. Despite overwhelming scientific evidence, he recommended COVID vaccines for Americans who had already been infected. Dr. Anthony Fauci was the mastermind behind these extensive deceptions. His justifications range from blaming the public (now blaming the unvaccinated) to blaming politics, with the phrase "you have to change with the research" being used to justify his unpredictable conduct. Dr. Anthony Fauci's refusal to fix the HHS's flawed vaccine injury surveillance system exemplified inexcusable irresponsibility. The public was never given information on infection fatality rates or COVID risks depending on age that would have allowed them and their doctors to conduct evidence-based customized risk assessments.

Trust the Experts

The CDC, the National Institutes of Health (NIH), the Food and Drug Administration (FDA), and others worked with the mainstream media to quiet debate on crucial public health concerns. Dr. Anthony Fauci's life-or-death obsession with revolutionary mRNA vaccines, according to the authors, drove him to overlook or conceal effective early treatments.

Fortifying Immune Systems

As a result of Anthony Fauci's COVID-19 lockdowns, Americans gained an average of two pounds per month, and their daily walks reduced by 27%. Zinc prevents and shortens the duration of colds by inhibiting viral multiplication. The World Health Organization (WHO) and the Centers for Disease Control and Prevention (CDC) have found that healthy adults with healthy immune systems have a minimal chance of getting COVID. Dr. Anthony Fauci's drugs and messages appeared to be geared to exacerbate stress and trauma. Our immune systems have all been demonstrated to be harmed by fear, stress, and trauma.

It's possible that COVID-19 was merely defanged to make it less harmful than the seasonal flu. COVID-related mortality might have been avoided in over 80% of cases if early treatment had been available. During the pandemic, taxpayers spent $660 million to build field hospitals around the country. McCullough claims that "therapeutic nihilism was the actual murderer of America's elderly." The number of mortality among hospitalized patients may have been reduced as a result of repurposed medications.

Independent professionals are currently administering treatment based on their best medical judgment and scientific evidence. Now is the moment to start healing people. In over 200 peer-reviewed trials, hydroxychloroquine (HCQ) was confirmed to be safe and effective against coronavirus. In monkey cells infected with SARS-Coronavirus, chloroquine has antiviral activities, implying both prophylactic and therapeutic effects. Dr. Anthony Fauci has worked to ensure that people with COVID-19 do not receive the drug hydroxychloroquine (HCQ).

In countries that allow access to HCQ, such as the United States, the death rate is one-tenth that in countries where this treatment is restricted. Most Americans are unable to obtain HCQ for early COVID-19 treatment, and even fewer are able to obtain it as a COVID-19 prevention medicine. Ivermectin was initially brought to IVM's attention as a possible COVID treatment. COVID deaths fell by 14 times in places where the Peruvian government properly distributed IVM. The Desert Review has called Dr. Tess Lawrie "The Conscience of Medicine"57.

In an urgent letter to British Health Minister Matt Hancock, Dr. Lawrie included her Rapid Review. The Cochrane Collaboration aspires to restore scientific integrity and consistent approach to drug development investigations.

Dr. Lawrie's speech should be remembered as one of the most influential in medical history. Big Pharma and other special interests, she claimed, have tainted modern medicine. Andrew Hill's ascension is just one front in the war between the NIH and the medical cartel to prevent doctors from using IVM. Bill Gates' foundation gave drug companies $125 million in tax-deductible donations. Anthony Fauci's drug Remdesivir has a catastrophic adverse effect.

The allegation that ivermECTin poses a lethal risk is described by Dr. Joseph Mercola as "pure horse manure." In NIAID human clinical trials, Remdesivir, which was developed in partnership with UNC-Chapel Hill, was proven to be efficacious against COVID-19. This is "a game changer," according to Dr. Ralph Baric, Dr. Anthony Fauci's gain-of-function guru. Vaccines can be dangerous and cause a condition known as Antibody Dependent Enhancement, according to Dr. Paul Offit, Merck's chief vaccine advocate. During a pandemic, a leaking vaccine "would put the world on a never-ending booster treadmill," warns Dr. Peter McCullough.

To ensure his immunizations gained rubber-stamp approval, Dr. Anthony Fauci stacked critical FDA and CDC committees with NIAID, NIH, and Gates Foundation grantees and supporters. Every virologist and infectious disease expert agrees that vaccines reduce absolute risk by less than 1%. By assuming credit for their vaccinations, Dr. Anthony Fauci and the vaccination business launched an opportunistic disinformation campaign. Official data on hospitalizations and deaths from the third wave of COVID-19 in Scotland revealed that 87 percent of those who died had been vaccinated. The COVID vaccine from Moderna has been connected to 7,537 cases of myocarditis and pericarditis in children.

17

The number of cases reported was at least 25 times higher than expected. Pfizer and the FDA may have agreed to call a halt to the company's study. This could be due to COVID. Those who have been fully vaccinated have 251 times the viral loads of Delta and other mutant variants as those who have not been fully vaccinated. Each vaccinated person has become a Typhoid Mary for COVID.

CHAPTER TWO

Pharma Profits Over Public Health

Anthony Fauci is the director of the National Institute of Allergy and Infectious Diseases (NIAID). Because of Dr. Anthony Fauci's clout on NIAID committees, he is able to get his pet drugs and vaccinations past regulatory hurdles. Under his leadership, drug companies organized the opioid crisis, making Americans the world's most overmedicated people. Big Pharma has a seamless extension in the National Institute of Allergy and Infectious Diseases. There is no space for error between the NIAID and the drugmakers.

The Office of Government Ethics admonished Dr. Anthony Fauci in 2004 for failing to manage the links between his personnel and pharmaceutical corporations. Dr. Anthony Fauci is in head of the $6 billion drug research and development budget at the National Institutes of Health. Under a secret, unpromulgated HHS policy, he and his NIAID employees might earn up to $150,000 per year from medications they helped develop. The GAO report makes no mention of Dr. Anthony Fauci's vaccine efforts for HIV, SARS, Ebola, West Nile Virus, or Influenza before moving on to commercial ventures. SIGA Technologies reports NIAID revenue but no royalties or commercial payments to the NIH or any of its programs.

The CDC sets outrageous retail cost for these collaborative items in secret conversations. Dr. Anthony Fauci played a significant role in Big Pharma's plan to destroy American health and democracy. He has turned the National Institute of Allergy and Infectious Diseases into a leading incubator for innovative pharmaceutical products, many of which profit from the growing chronic disease epidemic. Dr. Anthony Fauci has been chastised for recommending diagnoses and treatments that favour Big Pharma over public health. In every measure, his fifty-year reign has been a disaster for American health. On the other side, his commercial success has been infinite.

CHAPTER THREE

The HIV Pandemic Template For Pharma Profiteering

Anthony Stephen Fauci was born on December 4, 1940, in Brooklyn's Dyker Heights neighborhood. In 1958, he was the Regis High School basketball team's star point guard and captain. His heroes were Joe DiMaggio, Mickey Mantle, and Duke Snider. He is married to Dr. Christine Grady, the director of the Bioethics Department at the National Institutes of Health. In the United States in 1900, infectious disease mortality accounted for one-third of all deaths.

It has fallen to roughly 5% of all deaths in the United States by 1950. Experts feel that modern medicine played just a little role in the historic abolition of infectious disease fatalities. Vaccinologists have used vaccinations to claim a cherished and sanctified—and scientifically undeserving—status for themselves and vaccines that is impervious to criticism, questioning, or debate. By assisting state health officials in tracking down rabies and hantavirus outbreaks, the CDC was striving to legitimize its existence. Dr. Robert Gallo, Dr. Anthony Fauci's mentor, stated in 1976 that the CDC in Atlanta was facing downsizing and, in principle, closure. That year, government officials staged a fake swine flu outbreak, which temporarily boosted the CDC's optimism.

Dr. Anthony Fauci, according to critics, was neither a skilled manager nor a talented or motivated scientist. He got his first foothold by taking management of the AIDS epidemic from the National Cancer Institute, the Big Kahuna of the National Institutes of Health. Because Kaposi's sarcoma was the most common sign, the AIDS pandemic struck NCI. In 1984, NIH scientist Robert Gallo made the first link between AIDS and his virus, HTLV-III. In a debate with NCI's Sam Broder, Dr. Anthony Fauci persuaded him that AIDS was an infectious disease. By 1990, the NIAID's annual AIDS funding had risen to $3 billion.

The finance firm of Dr. Anthony Fauci has adopted political correctness as its new currency. When it came to HIV and AIDS, Peter Duesberg was not "wrong"; rather, he was politically incorrect. He vetoed every federal research budget after 1987 because he opposed the awakened viewpoint. True scientists were taken aback. Out of nowhere, a guillotine arrived.

A brand-new form of terror. "HIV denialism" and other "thought crimes" were "guilty." Thanks to Fauci, political correctness had become the new revolutionary language. And it meant you'd lose everything if you were "evil," if you didn't support agenda-driven science. The head of the National Institute of Allergy and Infectious Diseases, Dr. Anthony Fauci, is in charge of $7.6 billion in annual discretionary spending, which he largely allocates to PIs. PIs are a type of surrogate for the pharmaceutical industry who help to promote the pharmaceutical paradigm.

They promote ideology through their seats on medical boards and proselytize with missionary zeal. Dr. Tony Fauci and his pharmaceutical cronies rig the primary panels that approve and "recommend" vaccinations for children's schedules. PIs are obligated to approve virtually every new treatment they consider because of their financial ties to Pharma and NIAID donors. The "TV Doctor," Paul Offit, was a co-developer of the rotavirus vaccine that was approved by ACIP in 2006. Offit is a well-known private investigator for Dr. Anthony Fauci.

In the media, Offit is frequently referred to as a "vaccine specialist." Dr. Offit is the face of the pharmaceutical sector, its linked industries, and the chemical paradigm in general. He portrays himself as a reliable source of information, but in reality, he is a wellspring of industrial bullshit, deceit, and outright dishonesty. Dr. Offit is a member of numerous pharma front groups' boards of directors and has access to a wide network of bloggers and trolls. He voted to add Wyeth-Ayerst Pharmaceuticals' RotaShield rotavirus immunization to the mandatory schedule despite the lack of functional safety studies.

Dr. Paul Offit's rotavirus vaccine, RotaTeq, has caused a slew of catastrophic illnesses and excruciating deaths in babies suffering from intussusception. Despite the lack of true safety testing, ACIP voted in

23

1999 to mandate RotaShield, which was eventually removed from the market. Tony Fauci's decision to award pharmaceutical PIs practically all of NIAID's money for drug development was a breach of the agency's mission to find the source of the allergic and autoimmune disease epidemics that began under his watch. Pharmaceutical companies can divert federal funds to serve their own private business interests by using NIAID awards. It's no surprise that Dr. Anthony Fauci opposes non-pharmaceutical, non-patentable, or patent-expired medicines, as well as generics.

My paid speaking engagements decreased to one or two per year after writing an article on immunization safety in 2005. My scheduled presentations were canceled in droves by universities and business hosts that year. It marked the beginning of systematic censorship of any vaccine information that ran counter to official narratives. Anthony Fauci has been called anti-vaccine, anti-science, a "baby murderer," and a threat to public health by critics. Threats to disrupt money flows to university PIs take precedent over free speech norms. PIs at NYU attempted to remove Mark Crispin Miller and Mary Holland from their positions beginning in 2019.

CHAPTER FOUR

The Pandemic Template

AIDS and AZT

The AZT licensing procedure was a shakedown voyage for Dr. Tony Fauci, who would convert NIAID into a drug development powerhouse. AZT's lethal toxicity, according to a former BusinessWeek journalist, rendered it "so worthless" that he "didn't think it was worth patenting." To kick-start his initiative and provide legitimacy to his new administration, Dr. Anthony Fauci required a tangible accomplishment. AZT turned out to be a once-in-a-lifetime opportunity. As Dr. Fauci put it, the PIs were "out of control."

Because they were vertically integrated, they had complete control over the drug approval process. After three years and hundreds of millions of dollars, the NIAID had not developed a single new approved treatment. Dr. Tony Fauci was compelled to rely on Burroughs Wellcome's AZT and AZT-only agenda due to his administrative ineptness. The NIAID's lone arrow in the clinical trial quiver was AZT; trials were under-enrolled, and pharmacological treatments were never developed. Dr. Anthony Fauci's first reaction as the nation's AIDS czar was to instill dread of the disease.

He became a pariah among AIDS activists after writing a fear-mongering piece in 1983. According to the greatest scientific evidence, HIV's infectivity was so low that a pandemic could not last. In 1984, Dr. Anthony Fauci predicted that by 1996, there will be one billion HIV-positive people on the planet. According to the WHO, only 33.2 million people worldwide were HIV-positive in 2007. For years, there was a concern of catching AIDS through nonsexual contact.

Dr. Anthony Fauci was hesitant of exploring drugs to cure the numerous ailments that plagued and killed AIDS patients because of his concentration on a single antiviral, AZT. His efforts to sabotage therapeutic treatments were crucial to the establishment of the underground medical network. They claimed he was deceitful and dismissive of their concerns. Activists urged that the antiretroviral drugs Bactrim and Septra be considered "standard of care" in the prevention of AIDS. According to AIDS activist John Callen, the NIAID's refusal to fund trials on Bactrim, AL 721, Peptide D, DHPG, and aerosolized pentamidine resulted in the deaths of 17,000 people.

John Avlon's uncle, Senator Ted Kennedy, was the first presidential candidate to openly support gay rights. They spearheaded bipartisan efforts that resulted in the White House bean counters releasing millions of dollars. Ronald Reagan wants to turn over the whole AIDS effort to private pharmaceutical companies. Dr. Anthony Fauci disliked the fact that his office's expenses demanded separate budget columns that were not included in the massive appropriation from Congress. Rep. Waxman questioned why he never informed his legislative colleagues about the standoff, prompting a cascade of evasive and dishonest apologies.

He was dubbed a "murderer" and a "idiot" by Larry Kramer. Kramer compared NIAID to the group of miscreants, delinquents, and dimwitted knuckleheads from Animal House. "We lie down and die," Kramer adds, "and our bodies pile up in hospitals, homes, and hospices." Anthony Fauci's career was hanging by a string after congressional hearings on his drug-testing network. Only a sudden and unexpected adjustment in tactics might save his reputation and career. He instantly turned around and hugged AIDS activists, whom he had previously detested.

Dr. Anthony Fauci became a vocal supporter of "parallel track" approval for drugs like hydroxychloroquine and ivermectin, which are popular among buyers' club members. He questioned the ethics of FDA regulators who insisted on placebo testing of promising therapies during a global pandemic. Dr. Anthony Fauci implemented practically the whole ACT UP program at the same time. The AIDS community's network of 200 CRI doctors were testing anti-AIDS drugs in "parallel track" schemes with minimal expenses and quick enrollments. Big Pharma's front-line employees were openly rejecting his measures.

Due to Dr. Anthony Fauci's management style and his network of Pharma PIs, Parallel Track was doomed from the start. Teflon Tony designed AL 721 experiments to ensure failure and thereby trash the unpatentable medication. He'll use the same pretense in 2021 to destroy the NIAID's ivermectin trials. NIAID overlooked hundreds of additional effective medicines for opportunistic infections because "PIs have their own research agenda, which is not necessarily the same as the country's." Dr. Anthony Fauci manipulated key committees at the National Institutes of Health and the Food and Medication Administration (FDA) to control drug approvals by appointing academic and industrial scientists and doctors to the positions.

In HIV-positive patients who are healthy and have no symptoms, AZT has been licensed for usage. The FDA granted AZT an expedited Emergency Use Approval in March 1987. Dr. Fauci's team deemed the human experiment a success, and it was completed after four months.

A Moment of Triumph

AIDS patients who got AZT lived 10 times longer than those who did not, according to Dr. Anthony Fauci's AZT trial. He started his media blitz with an unprecedented move: he personally called key journalists at 10 a.m. to announce his victory. Anthony Fauci's remdesivir announcement was staged and tainted by fraud. He didn't have a peer-reviewed or published study, an actual placebo experiment, data, or even a press release to back up his claims. Using this fuzzy hearsay reasoning, he forced through Emergency Use Authorization for his favorite drug and sold it to the president.

The New England Journal of Medicine released Burroughs Wellcome's formal report on the Phase II AZT research, which provided the basis for FDA approval of AZT. The AZT trials were supposed to last 24 weeks, but Wellcome and Dr. Fauci opted to cut them short halfway through. Data manipulation, sloppiness, and departures from established procedures are all revealed in the documents. AZT is likely to cause cancer, according to an FDA expert who reviewed pharmacological evidence. Because of Dr. Anthony Fauci's decision to discontinue the studies, the inspectors were unable to investigate the remaining eleven facilities.

According to Dr. Lauritsen, the FDA's purposeful use of deceptive data is fraud. PIs covered up adverse events, violated protocols, and portrayed AZT patients as placebos on a regular basis. The FDA's Spitzig identified major discrepancies between the medical data and what the PIs stated on their CRFs. The PIs knew which patients were on AZT and which were on placebo, and they skewed the safety data in favor of AZT to give the AZT participants an advantage. "Many of the patients would have died as a result of the AZT toxicity if they hadn't been given emergency blood," Lauritsen, Spitzig, and Willner added.

29

To disguise AZT's terrible toxicity, Dr. Fauci used blood transfusions and other deceptions. AZT is the most dangerous long-term drug ever approved by the FDA. NBC News broadcast the first of reporter Perry Peltz's three-part exposé on the AZT Fischl trial, breaking the censorship blockage. Millions of people throughout the world saw the UK documentary, but not in the United States. By September 2021, Dr. Anthony Fauci will have mastered free speech in ways that have never been seen before in human history.

After pop sensation Nicki Minaj questioned whether COVID vaccinations could be causing testicular swelling problems, he hushed her with a simple word. The results of Dr. Anthony Fauci's much-hyped clinical investigations were less than stellar. In 1987, he claimed that AZT was 95% effective, claiming that 19 patients died in the placebo group while only one died in the AZT group. His long-awaited revelation came just as he was preparing a new whopper, which was ironic. The FDA panelists' significant concerns are reflected in transcripts of behind-closed-doors deliberations.

They were concerned that there was no means of knowing if AZT would benefit or kill healthy people. The intricacies of this momentous debate were only of interest to Celia Farber. Despite the fact that the suggested dose of 1,500 mg per day was entirely fatal, AZT became the "treatment" for AIDS. As a result of Dr. Fauci's fraud, hundreds of thousands of patients were persuaded to take

AZT. Many respectable scientists said that AZT was killing more people than AIDS.

Dr. Anthony Fauci had effectively given up parallel track CRI testing of low-profit repurposed pharmaceuticals by 1991. Instead, he used a loophole in the FDA's drug approval system to force truckloads of Pharma's new high-profit patent antivirals through. " Dissent was successfully repressed in mass-mediated public discourse. " Incorrect tests and epidemiology are utilized to inflate non-verifiable case and death counts in order to exaggerate the perception of an imminent calamity. To back up his favored approach, he's sponsoring and directing confirmation-biased studies.

collaborating with large pharmaceutical companies to provide them an advantage in the approval process. Tony Fauci, the director of the National Institute of Allergy and Infectious Diseases, has converted his institution into a profit-making subsidiary for himself and Big Pharma. According to AIDS activist Christine Maggiore, most aren't even aware it's a lie. It's more like business as usual than a deception.

CHAPTER FIVE

The HIV Heresies

According to Michael Crichton, consensus may be a noble political goal, but it is the adversary of science and truth. Science is disruptive, irreverent, dynamic, rebellious, and democratic, he maintains. The first to propose that HIV is the sole cause of AIDS were Dr. Robert Gallo and Anthony Fauci. No one has been able to create a study that can be used to back up their assertion with scientific data. "Today, the First Amendment simply does not apply to Tony Fufci," says Charles Ortleb.

It's worth revisiting Dr. Anthony Fauci's cornerstones for defusing suspicions about his subsequent pandemic mismanagement, particularly COVID. HIV does not cause AIDS, according to Dr. Peter Duesberg; rather, it is a "free rider" that affects high-risk populations. According to Gene Seymour, dissidents have raised legitimate concerns that should be acknowledged, debated, and examined. Dr. Fauci's zealous censorship raises suspicion and anger. Seymour: I'd love to hear those concepts discussed in a spirited discussion. It reminds me of George R. R. Martin's observation that established powers silence men's voices.

In Science Fictions by John Crewdson, Robert Gallo's daring flimflam, possibly the boldest, most bizarre, and most influential con operation in the history of science, is documented. Gallo is shown to be a mountebank who built a fortune by stealing other scientists' ideas and claiming them as his own in the book. In 1984, Dr. Jerome Gallo claimed to have discovered the root of AIDS. He persuaded HHS Secretary Margaret Heckler to provide credibility and weight to his bold announcement. In 1975, Dr. Paul Gallo claimed to have found a leukemia-causing human retrovirus.

Instead of being awarded the Nobel Prize for his discovery, he became a laughingstock once it was proven by other researchers that he had developed a monkey from the HL-23 virus. Gallo utilized a series of deceptions to make it look like two viruses existed, delaying the WHO's response by two years. Bob Gallo's work linking leukemia and HIV came dangerously close to costing him his job. Nobel Laureate Kary Mullis: In the rain forest or in Haiti, HIV did not come out of nowhere. It just so happened to land in [Gallo's] hands at a moment when he needed a new employment.

Gallo, like Dr. Anthony Fauci, has the National Institutes of Infectious Diseases (NIIs) and the press in his pocket. The NIH's legendary position helped Gallo's near-religious influence. Dr. Anthony Fauci's single pathogen theory of AIDS received all federal funding. Thanks to the "little emperor," NIAID became the go-to agency for AIDS research funding. He stifled any study into a multi-factor explanation by wielding his great power.

AIDS was a deadly disease. Dr. Francis Fauci's opportunistic PIs described AIDS as an amorphous disease with constantly changing criteria. HIV has infected 78 million people and killed 39 million, according to WHO estimates. HIV now affects 35 million individuals worldwide, with more than 2 million new infections emerging each year. Antibody testing for HIV are too expensive to be widely used in Africa.

The majority of HIV-positive Africans were asymptomatic. Women account for 59 percent of AIDS cases in Africa, whereas heterosexuals account for 85 percent. No one has yet explained how a disease that primarily affects gay men in the West might also harm female heterosexuals in Africa. In Africa, AIDS is nearly always diagnosed as a presumptive diagnosis because no 'positive' HIV test results are available. The easy option is to return to New York, where no doctor would ever diagnose you with AIDS merely on the basis of your symptoms.

Robert Gallo claimed in 1984 that he had "discovered" the HIV virus. In 72 percent of the AIDS patients Dr. Luc Montagnier tested, he found HIV proof. There are 182,000 persons in the US who haven't been diagnosed with AIDS but would be if they moved to Canada. Dr. Anthony Fauci threatened journalists in 1989 if they published Peter Duesberg's theory that the HIV virus causes AIDS on its own. Instead of using traditional methods for identifying sickness, he recommended doctors to conduct blood tests on both healthy and sick persons.

Science became prohibitively expensive without the financial support of Big Pharma and Big Government. The self-interests of the researcher, the research institution, and the biotech corporation all collided.

Antibody testing for HIV can discover proteins that are considered to be HIV-specific but aren't. The genomic sequences of viruses can be detected by tests, but not the viruses themselves. "It's not even a test for HIV," said Kary Mullis, the creator of the DNA amplification technology. In 1986, the FDA issued a warning that HIV antibody tests were not designed to detect HIV. Dr. Anthony Fauci's $15 billion HIV vaccine business flips accepted immunology on its head.

"What is the purpose of the HIV vaccine?" one could inquire. Both Sanger and Mullis asserted that HIV has never been isolated and that CD4+ "helper T cell" levels are erroneous. The failure of the HIV/AIDS hypothesis is one of Dr. Fauci's most perplexing issues. People who are not infected with HIV can be affected by any of the thirty diseases now known as AIDS. If HIV is the only cause of AIDS, this should not be possible.

Dr. Anthony Fauci's carefully prepared HIV-only theology was shattered during the 1992 Amsterdam AIDS Conference. Conferees saw the public statement as permission to discuss the formerly taboo subject of AIDS patients who did not have HIV. The CDC director flew out on Air Force 2 to Andrews Air Force Base to put down the insurgency. Dr. Anthony Fauci was seeking to portray himself as an open-minded scientist at the AIDS conference in Amsterdam. Dr. Louis Duesberg discovered almost 4,000 reported AIDS cases with no indication of HIV or HIV antibodies in peer-reviewed scientific literature.

In 1992, Dr. Tony Fauci declared undiagnosed AIDS cases to be a new illness. To avoid being accused of having Chronic Fatigue Syndrome, he named his "new disease" "idiopathic CD4+ lymphocytopenia" (CFS). According to Newsday, two of the "non-HIV AIDS" patients had Chronic Fatigue Syndrome. Dr. Anthony Fauci's thin skin, according to Dr. Peter Ostrom, who appeared on "Larry King Live" with Dr. Anne Schmitz and others, gets him into trouble. According to Harvey Bialy, the vast majority of HIV-positive people live a long and healthy life.

Dr. Anthony Fauci's actions effectively put a year's worth of work by about 100 independent scientists to a stop. One of the main goals of the study was to figure out why some HIV-positive patients do not get AIDS. It was a form of revenge against young scientists who dared to call for science-based funding.

All attempts by HIV/AIDS supporters to meet Koch's postulates, according to Duesberg, have failed. He claims that no one has yet been able to generate AIDS in a healthy experimental animal by injecting the grown bacterium. The only way to prove that HIV causes AIDS, according to Duesberg, is to demonstrate it in an animal model. Many HIV/AIDS campaigners were apoplexed when a study published in the Journal of the American Medical Association (JAMA) in 2006 shook the foundations of the previous decade of AIDS science to their core. Dr. Anthony Fauci has never explained why the viral load of HIV is always highest in the first few days following infection.

According to a study published in The Lancet, reduced "viral load" did not "translate into a decline in mortality" for people taking AIDS treatment combinations. Depending on how long AIDS patients live, Dr. Fauci supports the use of AZT and other chemotherapy combinations for months or years. HIV, according to UC AIDS expert Dr. Jay A. Levy, MD, is a time-bomb virus that remains latent in the body until it changes its genetic structure and turns into a fast-growing, aggressive, and fatal virus for unknown and unexplained causes. The CDC's annual estimates of how many Americans are infected with HIV remained remarkably constant at roughly one million between 1986 and 2019. The spread of HIV in Africa and the West defies the laws of viral pandemic transmission that have governed viral pandemic transmission throughout history.

AIDS' core of homosexual men and drug addicts has never been able to break free. Greene: It's confusing that AIDS does not spread to women through sexual contact. He claims that this is only additional proof that HIV is "just an innocent bystander or a passenger virus." In 2004, Reinhard Kurth of the Robert Koch Institute declared, "We don't exactly know how HIV causes disease." Robert Root-Bernstein, a physiologist, declared in 1987 that HIV is not the single or even the predominant cause of "AIDS."

In America's Doctor, Anthony Fauci's role as a high priest of orthodoxy who supports multibillion-dollar global industry is detailed. The evidence that AZT or subsequent antivirals reduce mortality rates has never been shown by America's Doctor. Demanding that proof is logical, though not hazardous.

CHAPTER 6

Burning The HIV Heretics

Dr. Anthony Fauci: Journals have devolved into knowledge laundering operations for the pharmaceutical business. He believes that pharmaceutical companies fund peer-reviewed journals, and that findings that question the Pharma paradigm are rarely published. The letter was signed by almost 2,600 people, including three Nobel Laureates and 188 PhDs. Thanks to Dr. Tony Fauci's loosening purse strings, the HIV gold rush had begun. The National Institutes of Health substantially funded Peter Duesberg's virology and cancer studies.

Retroviruses are responsible for the acquisition of many of our genes, and up to 10% of our DNA is retroviral. Duesberg's discovery of the first cancer-causing gene in 1970 inspired a new field of cancer research with his "mutant gene theory." For eighteen months, Duesberg read every scholarly article on HIV and AIDS. He disproved the hypothesis that retroviruses cause leukemia, cancer in general, and AIDS (the cellular opposite of leukemia) Duesberg's paper, the reigning father of retrovirology, was a masterpiece. HIV, according to Duesberg, is unable to cause cancer or AIDS.

HIV is a disease-free passenger virus that has coexisted with humans without causing illness for thousands of years. In the late 1990s, many teams of professional scientists began working on decoding the Human Genome. "This is the most compelling evidence that Peter Bialy has been completely correct for the past two decades," says Peter Bialy. According to Nobel Laureate Kary Mullis, Bob Gallo's identification of the underlying cause of thirty diseases in the United States and Europe defied common sense. Duesberg's contention that HIV alone can cause AIDS after 30 years has been cautiously accepted by most virologists.

Dr. Tony Fauci is one of the few exceptions. According to the Perth Group, Gallo's claim was absolutely incorrect. Dr. Anthony Fauci's entire career has been based on the belief that HIV is the only cause of AIDS. NIAID was able to pull jurisdiction—and cash flow—away from NCI by blaming AIDS on a virus. The discussion became one of the most dramatic and deadly battles in the history of science.

Because of Dr. Anthony Fauci, Louis Duesberg was almost never seen on national television. Being seen with him was career death for aspiring scientists. The NIAID inquisition's official proviso was repeated by the media, diverting attention away from the mission of "saving lives." In 1987, Anthony Fauci was stripped of everything at UC Berkeley: government grants, graduate students, a working lab, and conference invitations. If it hadn't been for his tenured position, Berkeley could have done without the controversial researcher.

Duesberg's appeal to the National Institutes of Health about the termination of his grant was denied. Tony Fauci argues that "the evidence that HIV causes AIDS is so solid that it practically doesn't justify any dispute." It was a secularized form of the notion of papal infallibility, according to John Sutter.

"I'm tired of hearing AIDS experts claim that they're 'too busy saving lives' to argue Peter Duesberg's points," adds Harvey Bialy. "Critiquing a dubious concept would divert time from more productive efforts," Dr. Anthony Fauci argues. In 2009, for documentary director Brent Leung's feature-length film on the history of AIDS, Dr. Fauci agreed to a sit-down interview. The NIAID Director's COVID-19 interviews have a recurring theme of double-talking and duplicity that will be familiar to modern Americans. Tony Fauci's theory that HIV does not cause AIDS is wrong, according to Kary Mullis.

Duesberg's most unexpected convert was Luc Montagnier, the man who first discovered the virus. The inability of many researchers to generate a complete review of the literature is compelling evidence in and of itself. A variety of reasonable theories to explain the pathophysiology of AIDS have been offered by leading scientists. What is the next step if HIV does not cause AIDS? In the first generation of AIDS sufferers, Dr. Louis Duesberg, an inventor, stated that drug use in gay men and drug addicts was the underlying cause of immune deficiency.

43

In the United States, many of non-HIV users are losing CD4+ T-cells and getting the same ailments as AIDS patients. In 1981, five gay men in Los Angeles became the first to get AIDS. Amyl nitrite poppers have long been associated to autoimmune diseases. The males were promiscuous partygoers who preferred the "fast lane" gay lifestyle. They were reliant on an antibacterial prescription medicine pharmacopeia.

Poppers were a staple of the homosexual social scene in the late 1970s. According to studies, poppers are suspected to be the direct cause of Kaposi's sarcoma. Poppers, among other organs, can impair the immune system, genes, lungs, liver, heart, and brain. Dr. Anthony Fauci went out on a mission to put an end to all discussion on cofactors like poppers. The CDC shelved the Haverkos study and issued one of its signature phony science publications to "show" that poppers are safe.

The study was "totally bogus," according to Lauritsen. Burroughs Wellcome profited from both the development of AIDS and the subsequent poisoning of a generation of gay men with the AZT "Cure." Tony Fauci acted as a traffic cop in this feedback loop. He used his regulatory position to promote AZT while simultaneously squeezing its rivals. Kaposi's sarcoma was the AIDS-defining illness of the 1980s, and it could be the cause of a variety of cancers linked to menopause. AZT is a highly mutagenic medication, meaning it causes gene mutations.

AZT destroys bones, kidneys, livers, muscle tissue, the brain, and the central nervous system at will. It targets the bone marrow, which generates lymphocytes, which are blood cells. Kennedy: Prescription medications can cause more harm than the ailment they are meant to treat. AZT killed tens of thousands of Americans before less lethal chemotherapy therapies were developed. He says that AZT's efficacy against amorphous AIDS was unclear, and that it was responsible for deaths during the pandemic's first wave.

Rudolf Nureyev, who died in 1993 at the age of 44, refused to take AZT despite his doctor's advice. Arthur Ashe wrote a column in 1992 in which he stated his grave doubts about AZT. Dr. Anthony Fauci, according to John Lauritsen, is the father of the AIDS pandemic. John Lauritsen accuses Dr. Anthony Fauci of committing genocide on gay men and Black Africans. The evidence implies that widespread use of AZT in the late 1980s and early 1990s significantly increased "AIDS" death rates.

The CDC promoted the myth that tens of thousands of Americans died of AIDS or HIV in the 1980s and 1990s. Dr. Claus Köhnlein, an oncologist from Kiel, Germany, began treating AIDS patients in 1990. "The initial prescription medication was AZT, and we now know that the dosage was way too high," explains Dr. Hans-Joachim Köhnlein. In his Oct. 30, 2020 exposé, "The Other Media Blackout," Holman Jenkins claims that the medical establishment has failed "to recognize involvement in poisoning hundreds of thousands of human beings." HIV-positive patients who take AZT have a considerably greater death rate than those who do not.

The homosexual press ignored scientists' urgent medical warnings about the hazards of poppers. Letters from dissident scientists like Dr. Louis Duesberg were rejected by The Advocate, a well-known LGBT journal in the United States. Blind confidence in Saint Anthony Fauci may be the fatal flaw of contemporary liberals. Robert Gallo might have earned the Nobel Prize for his discovery of HHV6 if he hadn't stolen HIV from Pierre-Ambroise Montagnier a decade earlier. Many critics had previously assumed that HIV and AIDS were synonymous.

According to Charles Ortleb, Gallo is a textbook sociopath. He realizes that submitting to Fauci is necessary for his survival. HHV-6 was a crucial collaborator in the HIV/AIDS alliance, according to Dr. Duesberg. Several studies have confirmed the link between HHV6 and AIDS, according to him. The National Institutes of Health promptly cut Knox's and anyone else's funding for HHV-6 study.

Scar tissue has taken over the normal architecture of the lymph nodes. When you think about it, HIV may infect people for years—even a decade—before they get AIDS. Human Herpes Virus-6 was found in 22 percent of CFS patients and only 4% of healthy people's lymph nodes. Many researchers have identified CFS as an AIDS epiphenomenon because of the potential that it is linked to the AIDS epidemic. Dr. Shyh-Ching Lo, Chief Researcher in Charge of AIDS Programs at the Armed Forces Institute of Pathology, was one of numerous doctors baffled by Anthony Fauci's unique thought that antibodies specific to HIV should be a sign of impending mortality.

In 1989, Dr. Anthony Fauci discovered that HIV is only lethal when combined with mycoplasma infertans. M.I.T. Luc Montagnier and Dr. Lo argued in 1984 that HIV might not be the main cause of AIDS, based on Dr. Lo's concept of HIV's genetic cousin. NIAID has still not funded any research on Dr. Lo's notion of HIV's genetic cousin, M.I.T., 35 years later. In 1984, Luc Montagnier and Dr. Lo suggested that HIV may not be the main cause of AIDS. Instead of chemotherapy, they claimed that common patent-expired antibiotics may be used to effectively treat AIDS. Despite the fact that over half a trillion dollars has been spent on AIDS research, Dr. Fauci has not budgeted a single dime to investigate their idea 34 years later. HIV's high priests are strongly averse to the notion that they might be wrong.

To exist, the HIV/AIDS religion has always relied on moral absolutism. Dissension is equivalent to challenging the validity of science, which is why dissidents are excommunicated. Scientist Kary Mullis says: Today's science is comparable to Galileo's excommunication in 1634, when he was told he had to retract his

47

beliefs or risk excommunication. Fear, intolerance, and terror have all played a role in the public's acceptance of this logically flawed belief.

CHAPTER SEVEN

Dr. Fauci, Mr. Hyde: Niaid's Barbaric And Illegal Experiments On Children

Dr. Fauci, as director of the National Institute of Allergy and Infectious Diseases, gave broad approval for unethical human experiments that exposed both children and adults to dangerous drugs. The arduous path to FDA clearance for AZT in 1988 prepared the door for a multibillion-dollar influx of new HIV therapies. He oversaw a significant expansion of his organization's influence over scientific research and global health policy. The National Institute of Allergy and Infectious Diseases (NIAID) approved AZT in 1987 as a result of Dr. Anthony Fauci's shady dealings with pharmaceutical companies. The Bayh–Dole Act of 1980 gave the National Institutes of Health (NIH) the authority to pursue patents on medications generated by his agency's PIs and then license those drugs to pharmaceutical companies.

The National Institute of Allergy and Infectious Diseases (NIAID) conducted a series of unethical experiments on HIV-positive foster children between 1988 and 2002. Black and Hispanic foster children were turned into lab rats by the National Institute of Allergy and Infectious Diseases (NIAID) and its Big Pharma partners. This isn't some fantastical scenario. Children are given drugs that cause genetic mutations, organ failure, bone marrow death, deformities, brain damage, and life-threatening skin conditions. The BBC's Nina dos Santos spotted the mass grave in Hawthorne's Gate of Heaven cemetery.

A semi-circle of tombstones encircled the pit, each bearing the names of over a thousand youngsters. These toddlers were doomed, according to the NIAID, since they 'had AIDS.' Dr. Anthony Fauci's HIV drug studies were found to have infringed federal law, including failing to protect foster children from harm. Many of the children tested by the National Institute of Allergy and Infectious Diseases appeared to be in perfect condition and may not have even been HIV-positive. Sixty-six of the trials were looked into.

The National Institute of Allergy and Infectious Diseases (NIAID) has approved the exposure of foster children to drugs for non-therapeutic, exclusively experimental purposes. At least 48 AIDS research on foster children have been identified by the Associated Press in seven states. The experiments were carried out in the name of Dr. Anthony Fauci's failed endeavor to develop an HIV vaccine. The HIV vaccination research of Dr. Anthony Fauci exposed babies and toddlers who had never been exposed to AIDS to potentially lethal side effects. Solomon: NIAID's claim that their tests were "life-saving" was a deception from the outset.

Dr. Anthony Fauci's testing were much more extensive, encompassing "at least seven states" in addition to New York. The majority of foster children were African American (64%) and Latino (30%), reflecting discriminatory policies that are consistent with HHS's long history of medical racism.

As a result of Dr. Anthony Fauci's clandestine interactions with pharmaceutical companies, the National Institute of Allergy and Infectious Diseases (NIAID) authorized AZT in 1987. The long road to FDA approval for AZT paved the way for a multibillion-dollar surge of new HIV treatments. Dr. Anthony Fauci's HIV immunization research exposed babies and toddlers to possibly fatal side effects who had never been exposed to AIDS. The majority of foster children were African Americans (64%) and Latinos (30%), indicating discriminatory policies consistent with HHS's long history of medical racism.

CHAPTER EIGHT

White Mischief: Dr. Fauci's African Atrocities

The idea of a disease-spreading unwanted minority was a typical authoritarian soliloquy. Dr. Fauci's PIs concentrated on developing nations that lacked adequate institutional frameworks to protect poor people from the abuses of powerful pharmaceutical companies. The National Institutes of Health and the National Institute of Allergy and Infectious Diseases were conducting 10,906 clinical investigations in 90 countries by June 2003. During HIV therapy trials in Africa, Dr. Anthony Fauci's DAIDS team employed another of his lethal chemotherapeutic vanity items, Nevirapine, to disguise fatalities and injuries. He persuaded President Bush to redirect US foreign aid dollars to the valiant effort to eradicate AIDS in Africa. Dr. Anthony Fauci failed to inform President George W. Bush that the FDA had never approved Nevirapine as a safe and effective drug.

Many African governments attempted to profit from the lucrative business of sending their citizens to clinical trials, and Uganda became one of them. The breakthrough was hailed by the National Institute of Allergy and Infectious Diseases (NIAID) as its most significant win against HIV to date. Nearly all of the study's safety/efficacy recommendations were broken, including the most crucial condition in "dosing safety" investigations, according to researchers from the National Institute of Allergy and Infectious

Diseases. Dr. Fauci used a preliminary WHO approval to persuade President Bush to spend millions of dollars on Nevirapine. DAIDS disobeyed practically every medical guideline, including the standard informed consent approach for reporting substantial risks to trial participants.

FDA investigators in Kampala described horrible mayhem. A private consulting firm was hired by the National Institute of Allergy and Infectious Diseases to examine and audit the Kampala facility. The NIAID and Boehringer's Ugandan researchers missed thousands of adverse events and at least 14 deaths. According to their flexible rubric, clinical trial employees assessed "life-threatening" injuries as "not serious." They contended that no one had taught the NIAID/Hopkins local team in Good Clinical Practice.

Dr. Anthony Fauci had persuaded Bush to make African AIDS elimination his moonshot goal. Similarly to AZT, Nevirapine was too big to fail, killing both mothers and children. "For the Bush administration, it was a major humiliation," says Robert Farber, former director of the National Institute of Allergy and Infectious Diseases. DAIDS said in July 2002 that it would conduct its own "remonitoring" of the Uganda Nevirapine research, to be directed by Edmund Tramont, Dr. Anthony Fauci's top AIDS aide. Due to insufficient documentation at the location, the trial did not meet Good Clinical Practice (GCP) principles.

Dr. Smith's findings put the mission-critical project to license Nevirapine to prevent HIV transmission from mother to child in jeopardy. Dr. Jackson's research team had not been trained on how to report SAEs, and his team had not been tracking or reporting AEs, even serious ones. Dr. Anthony Fauci had unmatched authority over the US health-care bureaucracy thanks to his ability to launch a $15 billion health-care program. Tramont began tinkering with data sets in order to align the rest of the report with the new conclusion. He revised the safety review committee's "unfavorable" conclusion to "favorable."

Dr. Anthony Fauci's coup de grâ€TMs was the White House statement that Bush will celebrate the scandal-plagued Nevirapine project with a personal site visit. The US AIDS media branded Ugandan President Yoweri Museveni a "benevolent dictator." According to NIAID's Tramont, Dr. Fauci's alleged NIH boss, Elias Zerhouni, should present Dr. Jackson and his Uganda researchers with an NIH funding. This would enlist the Director of the National Institutes of Health in the cover-up, bolstering institutional resistance to a full-fledged investigation. Boehringer Ingelheim's application to the FDA to prevent HIV transmission from mother to child was never resubmitted.

Regardless, WHO began distributing this lethal cocktail to underprivileged countries around the world. "This was a crime against humanity, not a sensible and reasonable decision," Dr.

Fishbein argues. In 2003, an HIV-positive African American woman died during one of Dr. Anthony Fauci's Nevirapine medication studies. At the time, Joyce Ann Hafford was four months pregnant and the mother of a brilliant thirteen-year-old. She had tested positive for HIV after a regular test.

Dr. Fishbein saw the remark by NIAID official Tramont as a signal to follow NIAID's strategic cover-up. In 2004, Thorpe and colleagues announced that their Nevirapine study had been discontinued due to higher-than-expected toxicity. One of the most expensive investigations in the agency's history. Dr. Anthony Fauci and H. Clifford Lane received royalties for an experimental AIDS therapy they developed.

The National Institutes of Health (NIH) has spent $36 million testing IL-2 on patients all across the world. Dr. Fishbein's interrogation sent NIH into DEFCON 1. Dr. Fishbein was able to obtain emails and other documents that detailed the behind-the-scenes activities. In meetings with his senior management, Dr. Fauci's principal strategy was to fire Dr. Fish Bein while keeping the Director of the National Institute of Allergy and Infectious Diseases out of the splatter zone. In 2004, Dr. Jonathan Fishbein was demoted and assigned to Dr. Richard Kagan, whom he had previously accused of misconduct.

Dr. Fauci's ostensible boss, NIH Director Elias Zerhouni, declined to meet with him to explain the demotion. Dr. Anthony Fauci was fired in retaliation for disclosing wrongdoing in the Nevirapine and Proleukin programs. In May 2004, the NIH agreed to begin an IOM study into HIVNET 012 in response to political pressure. The Institute of Medicine, on the surface, appears to be a credible source of scientific data. The IOM has again again dismissed Dr. Fishbein's claims.

The IOM panel purposely chose a narrow scope of investigation, omitting NIAID's gross misdeeds in Uganda and Tennessee. Tramont's action was a bold show of disobedience intended at the NIH's congressional overlords. The MSPB reinstated Dr. Fishbein after determining that his firing was "wrongful revenge." Dr. Fauci continued to punish him from afar, with implications far beyond NIAID. He came to a deal with the National Institutes of Health to end his work, but the terms of the agreement are classified.

"The African women and children forced to take Nevirapine were the real losers in that war," Robert Farber claims. Dr. Fauci, he argues, constructed sham clinical trials, disguised enormous wrongdoing, and expertly navigated politics. According to Farber, Joyce Hafford, who died of an AIDS-related ailment, was "always on my mind."

CHAPTER NINE

The White Man's Burden

In 1984, Dr. Anthony Fauci immediately promised the world an AIDS vaccine. Delivering a functioning AIDS vaccine would be the most persuasive rebuttal for the Duesbergians. The federal government has spent well over half a trillion dollars on AIDS. A decade after Coburn's protest, Dr. Anthony Fauci announced that he had developed a viable HIV vaccine. While his vaccine would not prevent transmission, he predicted that those who received it would find that if they did develop AIDS, the symptoms would be much reduced.

In Paris the year before, Dr. William Gallo's HIV vaccine experiments had killed three AIDS patients. NIH scientists combined vaccinia and a part of the HIV virus to generate the preparation. Three of their 19 Paris volunteers got the disease "vaccinia," which is often fatal. The project was halted by the National Institutes of Health (NIH) because to transgressions by Gallo and his collaborators on both sides of the Atlantic. Dr. John Redfield and his assistant, William Birx, reported in the New England Journal of Medicine in 1992 that an HIV vaccine they helped develop and test on patients was effective.

Drs. Anthony Fauciy Gallo and David Redfield formed the Institute of Human Virology, which has received nearly $600 million in grants from the National Institutes of Health and Bill Gates. They appear to have spent the majority of that money on African-Americans to test failed HIV medications and vaccinations. Despite his well-documented history as a con artist and imposter, Donald Trump named Dr. David Redfield to run the CDC. The White House coronavirus task group, which was led by Redfield, Anthony Fauci, and John Birx during the first year of the epidemic, also backed vaccines. Their partnership would culminate in a new type of corporate imperialism founded on biosecurity ideology.

That initiative would result in unprecedented wealth and power grabs, as well as civilization-ending consequences. Microsoft was fined $97 million for racially offensive remarks in its software and discriminating against African-American employees. European officials fined Microsoft $1.36 billion, the highest fine in EU history. In exchange for Microsoft agreeing to share computing interfaces with competitors, the Department of Justice withdrew its attempt to break up the company. In the early 1900s, John D. Rockefeller saw a chance to benefit from his family's medical legacy.

As a result of Rockefeller's efforts, more than half of America's medical schools were forced to close. His father was a criminal who sold snake oil while pretending to be a doctor.

The "Miasma theory" focuses on nutrition and limiting exposures to enhance the immune system. Those who believe in the "germ theory" believe that disease is caused by microscopic germs. According to miasmists, infectious infections are lethal in impoverished places due to malnutrition and a lack of clean water. William Béchamp's germ theory holds that microorganisms such as fungus, bacteria, and viruses are "our great opponents in fight," according to Dr. Claus Köhnlein and Torsten Engelbrecht. The "War on Germs" supports a militarized public health strategy and ongoing intervention in underdeveloped countries.

In 2000, researchers from the CDC and Johns Hopkins University concluded that vaccines were not to blame for the substantial drop in infectious disease mortality. Dr. Edward H. Kass scolded his virology colleagues for taking credit for the dramatic decrease. Engineers who built sewage treatment plants, railroads, highways, and freeways, not doctors, were the genuine heroes of public health.

Gates and Fauci's combative approach to medicine has spawned catastrophic conflict. Nutrition and sanitation are pitted against vaccines in a life-or-death war for resources. Any fair evaluation of vaccines in Africa must recognize that mass immunization campaigns are part of a larger strategy. The Rockefeller Foundation's yellow fever vaccination killed a high number of individuals and failed to prevent the sickness. Hideyo Noguchi, the Foundation's star researcher, died of syphilis after accidentally exposing orphans without their legal guardians' approval with syphilis vaccines.

Around the world, the Rockefeller Foundation was the de facto authority on global illness management. From 1913 through 1951, its health division operated in over 80 countries. The RF steered clear of health-care initiatives that were likely to be expensive, difficult, or time-consuming. Instead, it focused on increasing access to emerging global markets for US businesses. Bill Gates' foundation's working strategy has been dubbed "philanthrocapitalism."

Gates leverages BMGF's charitable contributions to obtain influence over international health and agricultural agencies, as well as the media. Thanks to deliberate giving, the Gates Foundation's capital corpus had risen to $49.8 billion by 2019. Dr. Anthony Fauci and Bill Gates collaborated on an AIDS vaccine research project. By 2015, Gates had spent $400 million per year on AIDS drugs, largely testing them on Africans. Clinton squandered billions of taxpayer dollars on this failed effort during his presidency.

Dr. Anthony Fauci's status as Africa's foreign aid Golconda helped Gates gain access to African public health policy. According to a New York Times investigation, the National Institutes of Health diverted $1 billion from the entire NIH budget to Gates' global immunization initiatives. Bill Gates and Dr. Anthony Fauci's medical neocolonialism initiative was the tip of the corporate imperialist spear. Following the conclusion of the Cold War, Islamic terrorism and biosecurity supplanted communism as justifications for US military and corporate engagement in developing countries. According to Dr. Anthony Fauci's agency, the NIAID's most recent AIDS vaccine attempt failed in 2003.

Peter Lurie was referring to the Centers for Disease Control and Prevention's (CDC) well-publicized decision to leave Black Alabama sharecroppers untreated for forty years in order to study the disease's growth. In 2008, Dr. Anthony Fauci put an end to the world's largest human trial of an HIV vaccine. The Merck/NIAID researchers discovered evidence suggesting the vaccine raised the risk of HIV infection rather than prevented it. More basic research and animal testing would be required before a vaccine could be offered. Gene Gallo's HIV vaccine candidate clinical trials received $23.4 million from the Bill and Melinda Gates Foundation and government funds.

Dr. David Rasnick: Fauci's dilemma is that he has repeatedly said that the presence of HIV antibodies is sufficient to diagnose AIDS. The search for an AIDS vaccine has taken longer than expected, and various setbacks have occurred along the way. "If we had a vaccine that could protect everyone, we could stop the epidemic," says Dr. Anthony Fauci. The Bill Gates Foundation contributes $400 million each year to the discovery of AIDS treatments. Dr. Anthony Fauci's strength comes from his ability to fund, arm, pay, maintain, and successfully deploy a large and dispersed standing army.

The National Institutes of Health (NIH) has a $42 billion annual budget, the majority of which is distributed through over 50,000 grants that support over 300,000 jobs in medical research around the world. Dr. Fauci and Bill Gates hired the charlatans who fabricated the research that led to the withdrawal of hydroxychloroquine and ivermectin. After reports that the COVID-19 virus was undoubtedly the result of genetic engineering threatened to tarnish his rule, he deployed the handpicked elite of virology's officer corps. Dr. Francis C. Fauci was the only US government official on the phone with Dr. Hans-Hermann Andersen when he initially questioned whether the coronavirus, COVID-19, could have come from nature. The NIAID gave about $155,000 to the employers of four of the document's five signatories.

Bill Gates and Dr. Tony Fauci appeared together on the evening news and Sunday chat programs to promote remdesivir. "Things won't be restored to totally normal" until a vaccination is ready, Gates stated in March 2020. The Gates Foundation and the National Institutes of Health have just launched a $200 million collaboration. "We want to go big or go home," stated Francis S. Collins, MD, PhD, Director of the National Institutes of Health. Dr. Fauci spearheaded a multibillion-dollar government initiative to create new vaccines for twenty virus families that potentially trigger future pandemics. Bill Gates' HIV vaccine and antiviral program is probably the worst in a long series of Western imperialist schemes because of its continent-wide scale.

Frequently, these are self-serving, one-size-fits-all vanity projects that only add to the tragedy. By utilizing his money, Bill Gates has infected international charitable organizations with his twisted self-serving ideals. His $1 billion in tax-deductible contributions give him leverage and influence over the World Health Organization's $5.6 billion budget, which he mostly utilizes to benefit his pharmaceutical companies. "The WHO's independence is compromised when a major portion of the WHO's budget comes from a private philanthropic organisation with the capacity to dictate exactly where and how the UN institution spends its money," says John A. McGoey, Executive Director of Global Justice Now. Bill Gates launched the GAVI foundation, which has raised more than $16 billion in public and private funds, including $1.16 billion annually from the United States.

GAVI redirects foreign aid monies away from poorer countries and onto pharmaceutical industries. Western nations formed the World Health Organization and the United Nations to represent liberal values. Bill Gates has demolished the global public health infrastructure on his own. He has privatized our health and food systems to serve his own interests. The ability of the Gates

Foundation to influence public health policy is dependent on its ability to ensure that safety laws are weak enough to be circumvented.

Bill Gates' resistance to C-Tap was inescapable due to his ownership of the World Health Organization (WHO). As a result of Biden's equity drive, Gates was forced into the open. In the face of Gates' tremendous power and influence, the idea that global health policy should be driven by democracy or equity failed. Around 130 of the world's poorest countries would lack access to immunizations by February 2021. Only 2% of all vaccine doses have reached Africa, and only 1.5 percent of the continent's population has received vaccinations.

Bill Gates made a name for himself battling for Big Pharma's interests during the African AIDS crisis of the 1990s. He overcame Nelson Mandela in a hand-to-hand confrontation with pharmaceutical firms. Gates' selfless altruism puzzled the press and the public for two decades. Gates fought back by "defending the status quo and successfully interfering for the billionaires," he said. Bill Gates, Dr. Anthony Fauci, and others wargamed ways for overcoming expected Black resistance in several of the dozen pandemic scenarios.

HHS solicited the support of Black preachers, HBCU college deans, civil rights leaders, and sports icons like Hank Aaron to alleviate the dread of jabbing in the Black community. African leaders opposed to

Bill Gates' COVAX vaccine venture died mysteriously after criticizing WHO immunization policy. The CDC did not investigate any of these deaths, instead blaming immunizations. Almost all of these deaths prompted a major shift in public health policy, from skepticism to strong support for vaccination. JFK dubbed Lumumba the "George Washington of the Congo."

The Congo's vast mineral riches piqued the interest of mining companies from the United States and Europe. The CIA, among other things, ousted regimes in Ghana in 1966 and Chad in 1982. Such antics show that we, as citizens, must be wary of the periods when democracy may lose control.

"White Man's Burden," a documentary, exposes the terrible implications of Bill Gates' medical intervention in Africa. By directing Africa's foreign medical spending to his high-tech, high-priced, and frequently unproven immunizations, Bill Gates is killing newborns. The health outcomes in the countries that receive the most Gates cash are the worst. Funding for nutrition, transportation, cleanliness, and economic development has been slashed as a result of Bill Gates' obsession with vaccine-preventable diseases, resulting in negative public health implications. WHO, GAVI, and the Global Fund, which operate as ideological commissars, effectively enforce Gates' vanity priorities.

Bill Gates' performance metrics rarely incorporate improved health outcomes, focusing instead on the number of vaccines and drugs distributed. "The Gates Foundation's failure to support basic care as fully as vaccines and research is a blind spot," Partners in Health founder Paul Farmer claims. Bill Gates' Global Fund has made a $59 million investment in Lesotho to help the country reach its high-profit vaccination and medical targets. Dr. Tony Fauci and Bill Gates' obsession with AIDS is great for companies like GlaxoSmithKline, but it's a tragedy for Africans. The Gates Foundation has invested billions in Sub-Saharan Africa through the Global Fund to fund AIDS and tuberculosis vaccines and antivirals.

Hundreds of patients in Lesotho and Rwanda said their hunger was "so terrible" that it made it impossible for them to take their anti-AIDS medications. The Gates Foundation's giving habits reinforce the colonial infrastructure that continues to "call the shots" outside of Africa. The BMGF awarded 659 grants to nonprofit and for-profit organizations, with 560 of those grants going to organizations in high-income countries, primarily the United States. The expose by Piller and Smith on Gates' African trip is a relic from another era. Gates worked hard to weaken the once-independent press with tainted grants.

He gave media organizations like NPR, PBS, and The Guardian at least $250 million in grants. The BMGF has put a lot of money into "strategic media partners" including Poynter and the International Network of Fact-Checking Organizations. In April 2020, Bill Gates and Anthony Fauci made joint appearances on CNN, CNBC, Fox, PBS, BBC, CBS, MSNBC, the Daily Show, and the Ellen DeGeneres Show. Gates' net worth has increased by $22 billion in the last year, but none of the reporters mentioned it.

CHAPTER TEN

More Harm Than Good

Dr. Anthony Fauci and Bill Gates have been accused of leveraging the WHO's public health agenda to further their own personal vaccination fixation. Most drugs cannot be licensed unless they have undergone placebo-controlled studies. The best of Bill Gates' African immunizations are included on this list. Dr. Anthony Fauci and Bill Gates have never given evidence to support their claim that their vaccines "saved millions of lives." According to the limited studies available, virtually all of Gates' African and Asian vaccines result in much more injuries and deaths than they avert.

Bill Gates has made Africa his personal fiefdom, and he is the world's "biggest vaccine funder." Pharma's goals in Africa are governed by WHO rules, which encourage cooperation and penalize resistance. It uses its financial influence to compel African countries to embrace more vaccines. A big study undermines Bill Gates' claim that his investment in the DTP vaccine saved millions of lives. Health ministries all over the world must meet DTP uptake targets or face losing important WHO HIV and other assistance.

The study examined data from Guinea Bissau, where half of the children were vaccinated and the other half were not. Bill Gates' DTP vaccine, according to a 2017 research, may have killed millions of

African girls unnecessarily. Altruistic Americans who donated to Bill Gates' African immunization campaign were actually supporting a continent-wide slaughter of women. Pneumonia, anemia, malaria, and dysentery were among the illnesses that claimed the lives of the young women. The World Health Organization (WHO) has rejected studies that show the DTP vaccine has negative side effects while approving trials that show the measles vaccine has positive nonspecific side effects.

According to an expert study, the Mogensen and Aaby investigations are "superior in every area" than the Gates-sponsored Lancet paper. In 2001, the Institute of Medicine recommended that thimerosal be removed from all pediatric vaccines. Robert De Niro and I offered a $100,000 reward to anyone who could point to such a study. There was no one who wanted to take advantage of the offer. The National Institute of Allergy and Infectious Diseases' Dr. Anthony Fauci worked with Gates on a project to remove thimerosal from African vaccines.

151 African newborns died in the experiment, while 1,048 of the 5,049 babies had serious adverse effects like paralysis, seizure, and febrile convulsions. The World Health Organization (WHO) has withdrawn its intention to distribute a vaccine across Africa. In 2010, Bill Gates backed the MenAfriVac campaign in Sub-Saharan Africa, which left African children paralyzed. Fertility research in India was supported by the Rockefeller Foundation, which historian Matthew

Connolly describes as "American social science at its most arrogant." Bill Gates' father served on the board of directors of Planned Parenthood, which supports birth control and sterilization.

The Gates Foundation has the financial and political muscle to intervene in foreign countries with relative impunity. It is unaffected when the trials it funds go awry, writes John McGoey. Bill Gates' father founded the William H. Gates Foundation, which focuses on reproductive and child health in developing nations. Bill Gates' apparent comfort with using coercion and deception to get poor people to engage in contraception programs they don't want is concerning. Two well-established paths to zero population growth are poverty alleviation and women's empowerment.

Bill Gates declared in a 2010 TED Talk that he intended to use vaccines to reduce the world's population. Some have construed his statements as meaning that he was attempting to sterilize women on purpose. Gates has never shown that vaccinations reduce child mortality, and science does not support this assertion.

Bill Gates contributed $2.2 billion to the United Nations Population Fund, doubling the size of the Gates Foundation. Depo-Provera users in the United States are 84 percent Black and 74 percent low-income; according to UN data, Depo is rarely given to White or wealthy mothers or girls. Bill Gates' team disregarded US research laws by failing to deliver informed consent forms to the women who were given Depo-Provera. By manipulating and distorting study data, they fraudulently "established" Depo Provera was safe. Bill Gates funded a WHO study to debunk the HIV connection between Depo-Provera and contraception.

Melinda Gates announced a billion-dollar commitment in July 2012 as part of a four-billion-dollar collaboration with USAID, PATH, and Pfizer. Bill Gates intends to distribute Depo-Provera, a birth control drug, to 120 million women in 69 of the world's poorest countries. According to Market Watch, Gates' investment might result in $36 billion in revenues for Pfizer. Bill Gates and his associates are deceiving African women into taking Depo-Provera by lying about the drug's safety and efficacy in treating ailments that disproportionately affect African-Americans. Bill Gates' racist gibberish has been aided by the director of the United States Agency for International Development (USAID).

The thought that Bill Gates, or any other renowned public health authority, would use vaccines to render women infertile is dismissed as a "conspiracy theory" by those who defend him. According to skeptics, vaccines may have been spiked with a chemical developed by the Rockefeller Foundation to sterilize women without their consent. Despite the fact that the WHO has been developing sterility vaccines for decades, individuals who revealed them were penalized. Dr. Christopher Elias was the president and CEO of Bill Gates' non-profit PATH, which collaborates with pharmaceutical companies to provide vaccines to developing countries. The Population Council advocates the use of artificial birth control and abortion to reduce global population.

Norplant, a very dangerous hormonal contraceptive implant, was developed with the help of the Council. Rajiv Shah, the director of the United States Agency for International Development, has ties to intelligence services as well as the oil and chemical cartels. In forty countries, the IRC delivers "humanitarian assistance." The polio vaccine campaign was initiated in 2000, following a meeting between Bill Gates and Dr. Anthony Fauci, with BMGF committing $450 million of a projected $1.2 billion to eradicate polio worldwide. According to a UN investigation from 1992, abuse in family planning programs extends back to the 1970s.

The Bill Gates Foundation (BMGF) has committed more than $1 billion to promote an oral polio vaccine containing a live polio virus in underdeveloped countries. Because the virus can replicate in a child's gut and spread in locations with inadequate sanitation and plumbing, anyone can receive the virus via the vaccine. Dr. William Henderson counseled Bill Gates against fighting polio in India, but he did so nonetheless. According to physicians, a vaccine-strain epidemic of acute flaccid myelitis, formerly known as "polio," paralyzed 491,000 children in India. According to a study, Bill Gates' polio vaccine causes polio in youngsters and "appears ineffective in preventing polio transmission."

75

In impoverished countries, malaria, TB, hunger, and diarrhea caused by unclean water kill far fewer people. The World Health Organization (WHO) acknowledged that Gates' vaccines were responsible for 70% of global polio cases. The hundreds of thousands of people who have died as a result of Gates' acts are regarded acceptable collateral damage as a result of his apathy to self-evaluation. The WHO is providing "unprecedented levels of technical help" to polio vaccine programs in Nigeria, Pakistan, and Afghanistan.

The Gates Foundation financed clinical trials of HPV vaccines in India as part of Gates' push to boost the companies' dubious claims that HPV vaccines prevent women from cervical cancer. At least 1,200 of the female participants in Gates' study had major adverse effects, including autoimmune and reproductive issues. In 2010, the Indian Council of Medical Ethics ruled that the Gates Foundation had violated India's ethical laws. Professor McGoey argues that the girls were not told they were taking part in a research study and were instead misled into thinking they were getting "wellness shots." According to Andrew Wakefield, "Gates' strong backing for HPV vaccines (Gardasil and Cervarix) sparked claims that he was using immunization to target human fertility."

"Under Bill Gates' regime, vaccine corporate profits supersede public health," he claims. In India, academics and public health officials have blasted the government's hepatitis B restrictions, citing the country's low HCC burden. Independent scientists and Indian doctors have argued that vaccinating 25 million infants every year is needless. The World Health Organization revised its plan to include universal hepatitis B vaccine immunization for all nations. Bill Gates contributed $37 million to a $37 million experiment of mass vaccination with Hib vaccinations in Bangladesh in order to demonstrate the vaccine's effectiveness.

WHO, GAVI, UNICEF, USAID, Johns Hopkins Bloomberg School of Public Health, and the Centers for Disease Control and Prevention (CDC) all claimed incorrectly that the Bangladesh study demonstrated that the Hib vaccine protects children from a "significant burden of life-threatening" diseases. Dr. Puliyel: I'm Dr. Puliyel, and I'm Following the World Health Organization's U-turn, Indian health officials were forced to advertise the ineffectual vaccine. He asserts in a BMJ piece that India and other Asian countries are now legally required to provide the vaccine and increase Hib uptake targets. Bill Gates' Global Alliance for Vaccines and Immunizations (GAVI) and the World Health Organization termed the novel, untested, and unregulated concoction the "Pentavalent Vaccine" (WHO). The true motivation behind the ploy, according to GAVI, was to increase vaccine uptake for hepatitis B and Hib. In nations such as Vietnam, India, and Pakistan, infants have died after receiving the pentavalent vaccine.

Bill Gates and the World Health Organization (WHO), according to John McGoey, regard the deaths as regrettable coincidences or collateral damage. Bill Gates' vaccine obsession appears to stem from a desire to commercialize his nonprofit organization and obtain complete control over global public health policy. His food, public health, and education strategies, as well as his corporate links, may indicate a messianic confidence in his ability to save the world.

CHAPTER ELEVEN

Hyping Phony Epidemics: "Crying Wolf"

Detractors accuse Dr. Anthony Fauci of exaggerating global disease outbreaks in order to raise pandemic fears, advance the biosecurity agenda, boost agency budget, promote profitable treatments for his pharmaceutical partners, and expand his personal power. At both the CDC and the NIAID, pandemic hysteria became an institutional policy. The Fort Dix swine flu virus was the same as the 1918 Spanish flu epidemic, according to pharmaceutical companies and the National Institute of Allergy and Infectious Diseases (NIAID). Previously, H1N1 was regarded to be a harmless pig virus that did not represent a threat to people. Morris had worked in federal public health departments for more than 70 years.

Because of the problems with the 1976 swine flu vaccine, the Department of Health and Human Services decided to stop vaccinating 49 million Americans. The government spent $134 million on the swine flu vaccine. Injured persons filed a total of 1,604 lawsuits. By April 1985, the government had handed out $83,233,714 in compensation. Flu shots typically induce fever in children and pregnant women, according to Dr. Morris' studies.

Dr. Anthony Fauci is a rare scientist who has remained at HHS for fifty years by aligning himself with the NIH's pharmaceutical overlords. According to Dr. B. G. Young, the vaccine division's industry-dominated culture has driven away honest regulators. In 2005, Dr. Anthony Fauci revived the NIAID's 1976 swine flu script. H5N1, an avian disease, was the villain this time. Much like Chicken Little, he has been warning the world about the impending bird flu catastrophe since 2001.

Farrar was at the epicenter of the previous avian flu pandemic, which was prompted by the misguided belief that the virus could cross species boundaries. He was a key figure in Dr. Fauci's endeavor to conceal evidence of government involvement in the likely production of COVID-19. "This virus is behaving like a natural bioterrorist," says Robert Webster, a pandemic expert. The Bush family's favorite doctor has received a Christmas wish list from the White House, which includes $7.1 billion for American security. President George W. Bush stated, "No country can afford to ignore the threat of avian flu."

Dr. Anthony Fauci predicted in 2005 that a new strain of avian flu may be as deadly as the 1918 Spanish flu. The impunity provision provided a blank check to Big Pharma's greed and illegal profits.

By the time it was all done, the World Health Organization estimated that 100 persons had died around the world by May 16, 2006. In 2009, he promoted another another false outbreak, this time the Hong Kong swine flu. The World Health Organization's management of the 2009 swine flu pandemic was "seriously harmed" by secrecy and conflicts of interest with pharmaceutical companies. Five European and African countries were forced to purchase millions of doses of Glaxo's deadly pandemic vaccine after the World Health Organization declared a pandemic. Van Ranst is a Belgian virologist with experience in the pharmaceutical industry.

As Belgium's flu commissioner during the 2009 H1N1 hoax, he was in charge of crisis communication. Chatham House is a private think tank that caters to the globalist and business elites. According to a CDC study, flu vaccines are connected to miscarriage, especially in the first trimester. Vaccinated pregnant women had a two-fold greater risk of miscarriage during the 2010/2011 and 2011/2012 flu seasons. Significant conflicts of interest impeded studies that received fast-tracked approval without functional double-blind placebo controls.

Dr. Anthony Fauci's erroneous declaration of a pandemic in 2009, according to Dr. Andrew Wakefield, reveals "dishonesty motivated not by medical concerns but by political ones." Wakefield: Private cash or targeted donations from certain countries are increasingly determining WHO objectives. Dr. Anthony Fauci, the director of the National Institute of Allergy and Infectious Diseases, received a lift from fear-mongering media coverage in his push for a series of "vaccines to save America from Zika." His business partner, Bill Gates, invested $125 million in a startup that is developing an mRNA vaccine for Zika. The Gates/Fauci Zika fraud cost taxpayers billions of dollars, and their "lifesaving vaccine" died this time in a syringe.

Dr. Anthony Fauci and Dr. Ralph Baric received $726,498 from the Gates Foundation to help develop a dengue vaccine. The National Institute of Allergy and Infectious Diseases (NIAID) in Brazil conducted clinical trials that found symptoms of "pathogenic priming," an enhanced immune response that can lead to system-wide inflammation and death. In January 2018, Dr. Anthony Fauci told the Wall Street Journal, "We do not anticipate this will be a showstopper in any manner or form." Sanofi's Dengvaxia vaccine was cleared for use by the FDA in May 2019. Vaccines for the COVID-19 pandemic, according to Padron-Regalado et al., should address the risk of adverse effects (ADE) similar to those seen with SARS and MERS.

The authors express relevant issues about human vaccine development. Tony Fauci, the man in charge of the global response to the COVID-19 epidemic, could have initiated it. According to the evidence, COID-19 may have originated in a Fauki-funded Little Shop of Horrors in China.

In 2020, Dr. Anthony Fauci devised a March Madness-style disease bracket. In a field that included his large array of made-up diseases, Coronavirus came out on top. COVID-19 has finally been proclaimed champion. The doodle's date was March 11, 2020.

Dark Winter was part of a long-running effort by intelligence agencies and the bioweapons lobby to maintain public fear about smallpox. In the run-up to the Iraq war, President Bush sought to inoculate the American people with smallpox vaccines. Soldiers were still being vaccinated using a vaccine that had not been proven, was not licensed, and was fatal. In response to the anthrax scare in 2001, Congress passed the Patriot Act and declared war on Iraq. The war on terror has benefited tech companies by at least $44 billion since 2001.

According to a 2021 research, the Patriot Act spawned "a massive terror economy." The FBI's chief suspect, Dr. Bruce Ivins, allegedly committed suicide after the investigation was completed. The National Institute of Allergy and Infectious Diseases, led by Tony Fauci, and the Pentagon's DARPA would be the two main supporters of pandemic superbug research. The Pentagon stocked up on 80 million doses of Gilead's flu medication Tamiflu in response to Farrar's fictitious pandemic. According to a report presented to Congress in 2001, the Pentagon's process for developing vaccines to protect troops from anthrax, smallpox, and other exotic bioweapons "is insufficient and will fail."

In the United States, biodefense funding jumped from $137 million in 1997 to $14.5 billion between 2001 and 2004. The NIAID's biosecurity budget jumped from zero dollars in 2000 to $1.7 billion after the anthrax mailings in 2001. Dr. Fauci might serve as a go-between for the El-Hibris at the FDA, resolving regulatory concerns about BioPort's lab and product safety. The Pentagon's plan to vaccinate US forces had been scaled back, and the Pentagon's anthrax vaccine stockpile had run out. BioPort still had the sole military contract, and Fuad El-Hibri said he was ready to ramp up production.

The NIAID's biodefense funding increased sixfold between 2002 and 2003. Dr. Fauci's choice to link infectious disease to terrorism represented a watershed moment in pandemic response militarization. The Director of the National Institute of Allergy and Infectious Diseases dismissed indications that coronavirus lab escapes were responsible for numerous epidemics in China, Taiwan, and Singapore.

As late as 1997, PREDICT appeared to be a reincarnation of the CIA's Argus project, which defied the Bioweapons Treaty to build apocalyptic "bacteria bomblet" under the guise of USAID. Under the guise of USAID, PREDICT seemed to be a revival of the CIA's Argus program. Nearly a thousand new viruses have been discovered by USAID's PREDICT program, including a new Ebola strain. Michael Callahan issued a cautionary statement to Congress about the country's new commitment to gain-of-function research. Biological weapon creation and development is a dark science analogous to medicine. Michael Callahan called Dr. Robert Malone from China just as the coronavirus was starting to claim its first victims.

Callahan had been treating "hundreds" of COVID-19 patients in Wuhan's epicenter. President George W. Bush declared BioPort's Michigan lab a national security danger after 9/11. Because antibiotics are a more safer, more elegant, and more effective defense against anthrax, the El-Hibris anthrax deal was particularly foolish. The antibiotic used was Ciprofloxacin, a low-cost, widely prescribed drug that Tony Fauci recommended. To obtain lucrative BARDA-funded BioShield contracts while fending off upstart competitors like VaxGen, the El-Hibris cofounded a lobbying group.

With the help of its high-ranking allies, Emergent turned the National Strategic Stockpile into an exclusive captive market. After NuThrax failed to gain FDA approval, the government increased its order of Emergent's core anthrax vaccine by $100 million. He lobbied hard to increase the government's stockpile of ineffective and dangerous vaccines. He doubled the number of El-Hibris doses produced each year from 9 to 18 million and increased the price each dosage. The pharmaceutical industry praised Kadlec's brash style.

Kadlec was in charge of the department's response to the COVID-19 outbreak. The El-Hibris paid the El-Hibris $370 million for anthrax vaccines. The National Institute of Allergy and Infectious Diseases (NIAID) has signed a development agreement with Emergent for a plasma-derived therapy. Gates backed Novavax's approach, which uses moth cells to generate key components at a faster rate than standard immunizations. Remdesivir had no effect on COVID.

Dr. Anthony Fauci conducted clinical trials to demonstrate that it could reduce the number of days a patient spends in the hospital by a few days. According to the WHO's far larger investigations, the length of hospital stay was not reduced. The House has asked Emergent Vaccine Innovations to provide over all federal contracts it has received since 2015, as well as all contact with Robert Kadlec, the company's CEO (HHS). Vaccines with defects were shipped to Canada, Europe, South Africa, and Mexico in large quantities.

The challenge of how to maintain control over US and global populations during public health disasters was the subject of the HHS smallpox simulation in 1999 and the Dark Winter in 2001. In 2020 and 2021, these scenarios, conceived and tested by health professionals and spies in 2005, will become our collective reality. Cambridge Analytica, the infamous data-mining firm, was owned by the Mercers' Strategic Communication Laboratories (SCL) Group. SCL drew among of the largest crowds when it set up a high-tech propaganda "operations center" at the UK's annual military technology display in 2005. Following 9/11, pandemic scenario planning became a critical tool for power centers to coordinate complex tactics for imposing coercive controls all at once.

The "Milgram Obedience Experiments" of the 1960s inspired the psyop techniques utilized in the War on Terror exercises. A psychologist named Stanley Milgram was a key figure in the CIA's MKULTRA mind control program. The CIA collaborated on torture, obedience, and brainwashing studies with the National Institute of Human Health (NIH), bringing the agency even more humiliation. MKUltra's simulations provided a platform for key decision-makers to approve previously inconceivable behavior that violated democratic and ethical norms. Scenario planning is a potent instrument for brainwashing prominent political actors, the media, and the technocracy into adopting anti-democratic orthodoxies.

In 2012, the epidemic that had been predicted for years finally occurred. Peter Schwartz was commissioned by the Rockefeller Foundation to create a scenario report. In order to defend themselves from viruses, he predicted that citizens will willingly give up their civic and constitutional rights. Bob Schwartz cofounded the Global Business Network (GBN) in 1987 as a corporate consultant specializing in intelligence analysis. He was a driving force behind the establishment of Wired Magazine, which went on to become the go-to source for mainstream Internet news.

Saro-death has been condemned by both the United Nations and the European Union. Nicholas Negroponte's MIT Lab developed Wiwa's Mondo 2000 about the same time as the CIA's infamous In-Q-Tel program, which attempted to penetrate the IT industry and put Silicon Valley on steroids by giving advantageous terms and government contracts. The ARPANET, which later became the Internet, was created by the Defense Advanced Research Project

Agency (DARPA) in 1969. Wired rose to prominence as an advocate of "Neurodiversity," a sort of autism denial.

According to Dr. Timothy Leary, "the CIA's reaction to Mondo 2000." Wired is also where the similarly sinister transhumanism movement got its start. Top Silicon Valley CEOs endorse transhumanism, including Microsoft's Bill Gates, Facebook's Mark Zuckerberg, and Tesla's Elon Musk. Francis Fukuyama has labeled the transhumanism movement "the greatest threat to humanity." According to In-Q-Tel, "transhumanism is a repeating aspect in our investing approach."

David Schwartz, Salesforce's chief futures officer, sells a "vaccine management" software platform that allows governments to track, trace, monetize, and enforce vaccine compliance. Schwab sees a bleak future in which SARS-CoV-2 mutant strains continue to mutate, leading to a rise in death rates.

By 2010, the Fauci/Gates partnership had risen to the top of the globalist biosecurity agenda. The "global struggle against contagious diseases" was used to justify oppressive government and corporate engagement. At the Munich Security Conference, Gates stated, "A highly destructive worldwide pandemic will occur in our lifetimes." In 2017, simulations were run to simulate a coronavirus pandemic that would continue from 2025 to 2028. They were eerily precise forecasts of the COVID-19 epidemic three years later.

Bill Gates' SPARS scenario simulated a bioterrorist attack that resulted in a global coronavirus outbreak lasting from 2025 to 2028. The official summary, which is 89 pages long, is a wonderful piece of foresight. It explains what to expect and how to respond in the event of a plague outbreak to public health workers. In the scenario, Bill Gates and Dr. Anthony Fauci promote remdesivir, a failed Ebola drug, as the "Standard of Care" for COVID-19. In actuality, federal health regulators exploit the PREP Act to shield vaccine producers from liability.

According to social strategists, the news media and social media corporations are anticipated to take part in the coup d'état. According to the simulations, the Fourth Estate's role as a champion of free speech and democracy would be compromised. They also believe they can destabilize social media, which was once regarded as a means of democratizing information flow. Bill Gates' simulations use the concept of "total war," which encompasses the mobilization of whole populations, the destruction of global economies, and the abolition of democratic institutions and human freedoms. Like all authoritarian systems, Gates' gambit would involve some book burning, which Bezos would cheerfully provide.

Bill Gates and Tony Fauci were laundering money to support gain-of-function studies at the Wuhan Institute of Virology Biosafety Lab. I emailed bioMérieux's former CEO, Stéphane Bancel, in May 2021, to ask if he was aware that his company had broken its contract by failing to produce a working system. Bill Gates has warned that a huge and severe modern-day pandemic is "quite likely" to hit in our lives. Biological weapons of mass devastation, he claims, have become "easier to manufacture in the lab." Clade X models the immune system's reaction to a bioengineered sickness for which there is no vaccine.

The chaotic response to the 2014 Ebola crisis affected the simulation. The effectiveness of repurposed medications in decreasing or ending the epidemic is not included in any of the models. The initiative was designed to give "experiential learning" for Trump administration decision-makers, according to John Sutter. The show was largely a commercial for Moderna and mRNA vaccines. Moderna's vaccine has received a lot of funding from Bill Gates, and his foundation has also invested in the company. The simulations in the article were designed to recruit and train public health workers to carry out their goal through censorship, propaganda, and, if necessary, state-sponsored violence.

Robert Kadlec, a co-designer, was President Trump's Disaster Response Leader at the time. Some of the world's most powerful public health officials serve on the GPMB's board of directors. Kadlec had planned to exploit a pandemic to undermine democracy and curtail fundamental freedoms. In the Crimson Contagion simulation, a "new influenza" pandemic originating in China, designated H7N9, was imagined. COVID-19, like other air travelers, spread the deadly respiratory virus fast over the world.

Crimson Contagion's planners predicted every detail of the COVID-19 pandemic, from the paucity of masks to the exact death toll. The precisely planned palace coup that preemptively obliterated the American Constitution was their overarching retribution. Chemical and biological weapons assaults were simulated in four TOPOFF (Top Official) exercises. In Denver and Portsmouth, New Hampshire, the first of them simulated chemical and biological attacks in 2000. The second, held in 2003 in Seattle and Chicago, had over 8,000 attendees. Bill Gates personally performed four simulations of a worldwide coronavirus pandemic for federal biosecurity officials.

Among those in attendance were former CIA/NSA Director John Brennan, vaccine producer Johnson & Johnson, and public relations firm Edelman. Event 201 was both a signaling exercise and a "government-in-waiting" drill run. Dr. Anthony Fauci and Bill Gates devised a computer simulation of a global coronavirus outbreak that would hit the US just weeks later. The simulation, dubbed Event 201, was as close to a "real-time" crisis simulation as one could get. A coronavirus has been purposely developed to boost its virulence and transmissibility in humans in Gates' simulation.

According to Gates' screenplay, mandates would spawn anti-vaccine resistance, which will be fanned by Internet posts. The fourth Event 201 simulation dealt with public opinion manipulation and control. Dr. Tara Kirk Sell is concerned that pharmaceutical corporations are being accused of intentionally spreading the virus in order to benefit from drugs and immunizations. Dr. Sell has worked as a sort of "Minister of Truth" for the US government, coordinating attempts to suppress opposition by the US government and the World Health Organization. Event 201, a conference on social media and public health, was co-hosted by Anne Halton of the Australian National COVID-19 Coordination Commission, which imposed the world's most draconian lockdown and abridgement of civil rights in that country's history.

According to Adrian Thomas, Avril Haines, Tom Inglesby, and Matthew Harrington of Edelman, the Internet needs to be consolidated. When "rumors" began to circulate, Thomas recommends a strategy for dealing with the problems that will eventually afflict pharmaceutical companies. Information access, according to Matthew Harrington, should be aggregated on a worldwide scale (Edelman). Singapore's finance minister believes that by holding dissidents and cooperating with foreign governments on "enforcement operations against fake news," the government can set an example. "This is a chance for us to expose such circumstances," said Singapore's Finance Minister, Lavan Thiru.

Event 201, Bill Gates' worldwide pandemic war simulation, was reaching and indoctrinating its intended audience. Foreigners who questioned government orthodoxies about COVID-19 vaccines would be tracked, according to MI6, the British intelligence agency. Eavesdropping on or surveilling US citizens is illegal for US spy agencies. Germany's domestic intelligence service has announced that it will begin spying on the top officials of the group who invited me. UNICEF hailed the Maldives for passing a bill making it illegal for parents to decline any government-recommended immunization for their children.

The Wellcome Trust, a GlaxoSmithKline company, has played a crucial part in the Big Pharma-Western intelligence agency collaboration. Dr. Anthony Fauci and other Western health professionals have mentioned the Imperial College's inaccurate COVID-19 fatality projections. The New York Post and the New York Times, he claims, have been ardent backers of a strong pandemic response. The Post's new owner, Jeff Bezos, has done little to undo the CIA's corrosive influence. Bill Gates, Apple CEO Tim Cook, Mark Zuckerberg, Amazon CEO Jeff Bezos, Mike Bloomberg, and Google co-founders Larry Page and Sergey Brin.

The board of directors includes Warren Buffett, Netflix CEO Reed Hastings, Disney Chairman Robert Iger, and Viacom/CBS Chairman Shari Redstone. The CIA, Internet tycoons, medical technocrats, and corporate scumbags orchestrated the ultimate coup d'état. They shut down churches, companies, postponed jury trials for corporate crooks, and violated people's privacy with unwarranted searches and track-and-trace surveillance.

Operation Warp Speed, a $10 billion Defense Department effort with "strong military participation," is a well-organized operation. According to the flowchart, the effort is overseen by four generals and sixty other military officials. Health officials protested that they were being neglected as Warp Speed developed into a partnership between the military and the pharmaceutical business. Dr. Anthony Fauci, who described Operation Warp Speed as a "talent show," was unconcerned about the military's control of US health policy. Mohed Slaoui and Gustave Perna, respectively, are the CEO and vice president of Operation Warp Speed.

Former Special Forces veteran Paul Ostrowski is in charge of vaccination distribution. Matt Hepburn is a Pentagon researcher who focuses on cutting-edge military technology.

CHAPTER TWELVE

Germ Games

War Games: Genesis of the Biosecurity State

The military and the pharmaceutical business worked on bioweapons development during WWII. Frank Olson fell to his death from a window in New York's Hotel Statler in 1953 after being poisoned with LSD by a CIA colleague. When the US government admitted to being responsible for Olson's death, his family was offered an out-of-court settlement. The Biological Weapons Convention, which outlaws the development, use, and storage of biological weapons, was signed by the United States in 1972. Under the provisions of the agreement, anthrax and other biological warfare agents might be manufactured for vaccine production.

The peace dividend was never realized, and by 9/11, the Soviets had been replaced as the major adversary in US foreign policy. Robert P. Kadlec9 is an American physician and a former Colonel in the United States Air Force. He was Assistant Secretary of Health and Human Services for Preparedness and Response from August 2017 to January 2021, when he supervised the COVID-19 crisis during the Trump administration. According to Bob Kadlec's email, Dr. Anthony Fauci and others were gathering together material for the dubious official explanation that they would tell the world. Both men were involved in campaigning for and sponsoring hazardous projects under NIAID and BARDA.

He was named Special Assistant for Biodefense Planning to President George W. Bush after the anthrax attacks. His lobbying efforts were successful in persuading Congress to establish a biodefense industrial complex. Some of Inglesby's most notable investments backed a series of simulations he presided over at his Johns Hopkins Center. In the case of a pandemic, police powers were used to detain and isolate citizens during the drills. In 1998, a small group of imaginary terrorists produced a few pounds of anthrax for Pentagon anthrax research in Nevada.

Two years later, someone launched an anthrax attack on members of Congress and significant media figures. According to my uncle, biosecurity may eventually displace Islamic terrorism as the focal point of US foreign policy. Following the 2001 anthrax attacks, "vaccines" became a euphemism for the development of bioweapons. Military planners at the Pentagon, BARDA, DARPA, and the CIA poured money into "gain-of-use" projects. The El-Hibris' bankruptcy turned out to be their saving grace.

The Dark Winter experiment foretold many aspects of what would happen months later with the anthrax letter. Starting in Oklahoma City, the Germ Game simulated a smallpox pandemic across the United States. The CIA's presence was undeniable in this and subsequent simulations. Dr. Margaret O'Toole's zeal for germ warfare, according to specialists, affected her judgment. Dr. Michael Lane calls her smallpox transmission predictions "impossible" and "absurd," while Dr. James Fauci calls them "much, much worse than would have been the case" in reality.

The COVID-19 vaccination contracts were signed by Robert Kadlec, HHS's Chief of Preparedness and Response. According to records, drug companies demanded flexible supply schedules and immunity from liability if vaccines failed. The Dark Winter simulation predicted the anthrax attacks that occurred less than three months later. Hauer is an outspoken supporter of mandatory vaccines for employees. PNAC members dubbed themselves "The Vulcans" in honor of their brutal style of US imperialism.

Critics dubbed them the "Chicken Hawks" because they refused to participate in the Vietnam War draft. Carrie Miller's jingoistic reporting aided in the US invasion of Iraq. She illegally leaked the identity of CIA spy Valerie Plame in order to punish her husband, Joseph Wilson. For her conduct, Libby, who alerted Miller that Plame was a covert CIA operative, was condemned to prison. The fact that Libby was a part of the worldwide vaccine scheme should cause us to think twice.

The CIA was involved in at least 72 attempted and successful coups d'états between 1947 and 1989. Rather than promoting democracy or public health, it promotes authority and control.

CONCLUSION

There you have it - a complete summary of The Real Anthony Fauci by Robert F. Kennedy Jr.

As you can see from the book, Robert F. Kennedy Jr. takes on Bill Gates, Anthony Fauci, the media, and the pharmaceutical industry. He painted Fauci, the US government's chief medical advisor, as a villain. He claimed to be a puppetmaster, a powerful technocrat who masterminded and carried out the historic coup against Western democracy in 2020.

The head of the National Institute of Allergy and Infectious Diseases, Anthony Fauci, is in bed with Bill Gates and the world's pharmaceutical companies. According to the author, they intend to establish a powerful vaccine cartel that would extend the epidemic and exaggerate its devastating effects in order to market pricey vaccinations. The so-called mainstream media and huge tech corporations, which reportedly withheld critical news, are said to be backing them, as befits a conspiracy theory.

THE END

Made in United States
Troutdale, OR
08/14/2023

12045090R00056